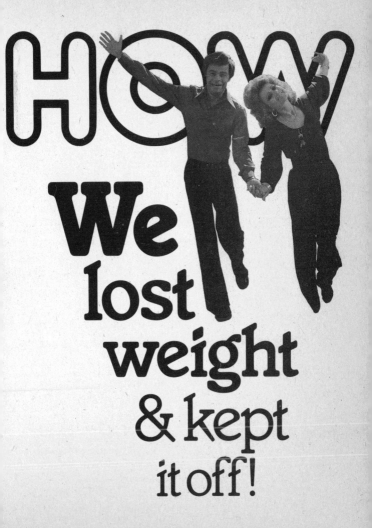

JIM & TAMMY BAKKER
with Dr. Stephen Gyland and Jeffrey Park

HOW
We
lost
weight
& kept
it off!

"Who satisfieth thy mouth with good things; so that thy youth is renewed like the eagles."

—Psalms 103:5

CONTENTS

FOREWORD

The writer of Proverbs says several times, "there is a way that seemeth right to a man, but the end thereof are the ways of death."

This is certainly true spiritually — but it's also true physically.

In our country and in our society, we have adopted so many habits that seem "right" to us, but are actually hastening our physical deaths. How many wonderful Christian men and women, husbands and wives, and even renowned ministers have we lost prematurely, because of ailments related to over-eating and lack of exercise? How many times have you and I been knocked out of commission and prevented from doing worthwhile things because our bodies let us down? Maybe our blame is misplaced — maybe we've let our bodies down!

Paul asks, "Don't you know that your body is the temple of the Holy Spirit?" And he also reminds Timothy that bodily exercise does profit — though he emphasizes spiritual exercise more. I truly doubt that the great men and women of the Old Testament, and even the New Testament, could have performed their wondrous exploits if they had been living on the kind of processed, chemical-riddled sugar coated diets that we do. Shirley and I firmly believe that the miraculous deeds of the Bible were most often a combination of God's wonder working power and His servants' best efforts. If it were true then . . . then it's true now.

I really and truly believe the Lord will be pleased if we take care of these wonderful bodies He's given us, and "look after the temple." Jim and Tammy have discovered a great many health "secrets;" actually, they're not secrets at all, but obvious truths that have been buried by the "progress' and Madison Avenue packaging of our society. Imagine calling a cigarette, "LIFE?"

There are so many ways that seem right to man, when their end is really sickness and death. We hope you'll benefit from the Bakkers' example, and grow with all of us, body, soul and spirit in Jesus' Name.

> *We love you,*
> PAT & SHIRLEY BOONE

INTRODUCTION

In the past six months, Tammy and I have experienced a wonderful rejuvenation in body, mind and spirit. Coming during a time of great testing at PTL, we have felt better than ever before, both spiritually and physically.

A principal reason is the diet and exercise plan that God gave us last fall. Since then, God has provided us a "complete tune-up" and our bodies are functioning so much better. It has blessed every area of our lives.

Because we believe that prosperity in health is God's desire and the inheritance of every Christian, we want to share our discoveries with you. As one who prays much for the sick, I am coming to discover that much sickness can be avoided through good nutrition, exercise, and proper care of the body, which is the "temple of the Holy Spirit."

The thoughts and ideas of this book are shared out of what we have learned from scripture and our own experience. While most all of them can be applied generally, body care must be applied individually with God's best guidance and good medical advice. We have, therefore, included comments from a wonderful, dedicated Christian physician, Stephen Gyland of Jacksonville, Florida. Doctor Gyland is a leader in his field. We deeply love and respect this man of God and thank him for his comments. We suggest you may also consult your own physician.

We also want to thank our own staff writer, Jeff Park, who organized and researched much of the material in this book.

Finally, we pray that you will be blessed with a new vigor for life and God's service as you read and join us in rediscovering God's best for our whole beings.

In warmest Christian love,

Jim & Tammy Bakker

HOW
We lost
weight
& kept
it off!

Jeff: **Jim and Tammy, I know that you have been dieting for several months now, how and why did you start?**

Tammy: A friend of mine at PTL, Beverly Wright, came up to me one day and said, "Tammy, you and I need to go on a diet together." I was shocked! I knew I was overweight — 130 pounds which is too much for my 4′ 10½″ frame. But I wore loose fitting clothes so I didn't think my weight problem was so obvious to everyone else. I decided then and there I must do something.

Jim: It started with my around the world mission trip. During the first part of the trip, the food was excellent. The Oriental people have wonderful food. They concentrate on rice and vegetables cooked with little or no water to keep in nutrients. Their meat is mostly poultry and fish. As a result, they are very healthy people.

However, when we got to India and Africa the food was difficult to eat. I ate very lightly. In addition, the itinerary was very strenuous, physically. Some days we walked several miles with our luggage to and from airplanes. Instead of feeling exhausted, I felt better than ever. I found I didn't need to eat so much and the physical exercise was exhilarating.

Jeff: **Dr. Gyland, why should one go on a diet?**

Doctor   That is mostly an individual question. I en-
Gyland: counter people that want to diet for practically every reason under the sun. The motivation of my wife's dieting is different than mine. But I believe the best reason that a person should diet is for good health — to take better care of their body, which is the Temple of the Holy Spirit according to God's Word (I Corinthians 3:16).

Jeff: **Your reasons, then were primarily to lose weight?**

Tammy: Yes, at least at first. It wasn't that being overweight was hindering me that much spiritually or physically. I really didn't like the way I looked, being so heavy. However, I do have weak knees and last winter, going up stairs was real hard. I even had to wear knee braces. Being overweight added a lot to that problem.

Jim: Actually, it was more that I felt healthier, than it was that I wanted to lose weight. When I returned from the world trip, I was several pounds lighter and I saw that Tammy had lost weight, too. We decided to continue our efforts in dieting and exercise together. Also, I felt so good physically and I wanted to keep that up. Right then, PTL was having financial difficulties and a telethon was upcoming. I knew I would need all the physical strength possible to do my best. This was my incentive at the start.

Jeff: **Had you tried dieting before?**

Tammy: Yes, a couple of times. When I got married, I was tiny — weighed only 83 pounds. But then I wasn't fully developed as a woman. After a number of years on the evangelistic field, both Jim and I gained weight because of irregular eating and staying in pastor's homes where we were often treated to rich Sunday dinners. One time we decided that we had to do something so we determined we would cut out all sweets and not eat any desserts.

We didn't know how to go about dieting right. After a week or so we got such a craving for sweets that when we passed a bakery and saw this beautiful chocolate cake in the window, we went and bought it and took it back to the motel and ate the whole thing. That destroyed our thoughts of dieting for awhile.

Another time, after Tammy Sue was born, I lost a lot of weight. But it wasn't by dieting. I was so emotionally troubled that I couldn't enjoy eating anything. So even at my proper weight, I didn't feel whole inside.

Jim: Yes, I have tried often — most of the time out of guilt and it never lasted. When I say guilt, I mean reacting to people's comments. I have been a little overweight for a number of years. And television is very unkind in portraying a person's weight. Often when I would meet a person for the first time who had seen me on the air, they'd comment, "Why, you don't look as fat in person as on TV." Comments like that would hurt and I'd try to diet. But I had no real vision about diet and good health before. Unfortunately, most people today diet out of guilt and negative reasons so they don't find lasting results and satisfaction.

Jeff: **Do you feel that the Lord has to impress one to diet?**

Tammy: Not really. I'm sure it gives one incentive and strength if God speaks to your heart. But God clearly says in His Word that we are to take care of our bodies. That includes overeating.

Jim: No. But in actuality if we read our Bible, He already has. Our American society has a way of playing up certain sins like murder, robbery and adultery, but playing down others like gossip and gluttony. We basically live in a gluttonous society so we tend to ignore it. God's penalty for gluttony in the Old Testament was the same as murder — death by stoning (Deut. 21:20, 21). In murder, you kill someone else; gluttons kill themselves.

God's standards haven't changed. Jesus placed gluttons in the same category as drunkards. Addiction to food can be as spiritually harmful as addiction to alcohol.

But God's Word concerning food and eating is far from all negative. One of my favorite promises in the Bible is Psalms 103, verse 5: "He satisfies my mouth with good things, so my youth is renewed like the eagles." This is God's promise. The key to understanding this is to know what are good things. Many of us think that good things are only those that taste good like sweets. But in Christ, even our taste buds must be redeemed. The good things are those that God created ("It is good"). He will show us, if we seek Him, the good things to eat, so that we can have a healthy and renewed body — strong for His service.

The testimony of the prophet Daniel while in training for service in the courts of the Media-Persian empire, verifies this. God showed Daniel the diet of vegetables and water was better than the rich, spicy and wine-filled diet of the Medes. God rewarded Daniel's obedience to the vegetable diet with better health and a greater alertness, mentally and spiritually.

These same rewards are available to us. If we will commit our exercise and eating habits to God and trust in His guidance, He will bless us with better health and mental and spiritual alertness. (See Appendix I for God's promises to dieters.)

Jeff: **What did you do to get started on your diet?**

Tammy: I began to watch what I ate and reduced my food intake. But most important to me was exercise. I am short, so much of my weight settled in my tummy and hips. I could actually knead my stomach like dough. It was that bad. I knew the flabby tummy and hips were not going to go away just by eating less.

Jim: I was already on my diet because of the strange food in India and Africa before I really knew it. When I got back to the States, I was already feeling better and healthier. I determined to keep my food intake lower and keep myself in shape physically with exercise.

Doctor   The first thing I do in starting a person on a diet is
Gyland: to have them honestly face the facts of what they are eating and what it is doing to their body. As Jim has said we live in a gluttonous society. Gluttony as sin takes its toll in heart diseases, hardening of the arteries and probably some cancer — most of the major causes of death in America.

If a person is overweight, he needs to face it and make a decision to correct it. One can easily see approximately what their weight should be based on their height and frame by checking a weight chart. (See Appendix II.)

I must point out that not all overweight persons are gluttonous. Many overweight persons just have their thermostat (set for weight instead of temperature) set too high, and they actually eat less food or food may be less important to them than to people who by genetics or activity are thin by nature. The fat person who is not gaining weight is not eating any more calories than the thin person who is also stable at his weight. However, whether or not the fat person really suffers from gluttony, for the benefit of his own health, well being and longevity and his Christian witness, he should trim down to a more reasonable weight even though it means eating less calories than the thin person has the pleasure of eating.

When a person really makes a firm decision in their heart to lose weight, almost always a way to accomplish that can be found. The solution will be different for different people according to their particular metabolism. The greatest problem that I, and many of my patients, have in dieting is keeping my eyes on the solution and not looking back. If we let our minds dwell on all those "goodies" that caused our problems, just like Lot's wife did and the Israelites did in the wilderness, we will never get victory over our problem.

Jeff: **You feel that dieting and exercise are intertwined?**

Tammy: Definitely. They both have to do with how we take care of our bodies which is the temple of our soul and spirit. If one is dieting primarily to lose weight, proper exercise is especially important. I've never been a disciplined person, I've always just struggled to get to know "me" and who I am. That includes deciding what I choose to eat and also how I keep my body in shape.

Jim: Yes. They both have to do with a healthy body — which strongly affects our mental and spiritual attitudes. Health is my goal and purpose in both proper eating habits and physical exercise. Diet and exercise are interrelated in that my eating habits affect my body agility and exercise affects my body's desire for food.

Doctor   Certainly, dieting and exercise are interrelated.
Gyland: The greatest value of exercise is to allow a person to feel better. The more you exercise the more alive you feel.

         If you don't exercise any, you won't have the energy to do other things you may want to do. Those who don't exercise are likely to feel tired so they want to eat because they've experienced before that food gives them energy. That may or may not be the case in a particular situation. You may be tired because of obesity, and eating is not going to help.

Jeff: **Can one effectively diet or exercise without doing both?**

Tammy: Not effectively! Dieting still leaves you flabby and most bulges don't go away with just dieting. On the other hand I don't feel that exercise takes off that much weight, especially trouble weight. However, with exercise and diet you have a winning combination. You lose pounds and bulges.

Jim: I think that a person can concentrate on one or the other. But if a person either diets or exercises effectively, he or she will find the one affecting the other. And in doing either, it can be done better with the other.

Doctor Gyland: I always encourage exercise along with dieting — not only as a way to better health but also to lose weight. It takes about an hour of continuous jogging to burn off just 500 calories, but more importantly as a sedentary, obese person begins to increase his exercise, he has a markedly decreased desire for food. So the total calorie loss of the extra calories burned added to the extra calories that are no longer eaten results in a very nice weight loss.

It might be pointed out at this point that more important than just losing weight is losing fat. As a person not only diets but exercises, he begins to burn up his fat and may actually increase his bone and muscle tissue. This doesn't show as much weight loss but produces a better-looking, healthier body. When thin people increase their exercising, it makes them healthier, also. Although they don't experience the loss of weight, they do have the physical well being and increase in muscle and bone tissue.

Jeff: **What kind of exercises do you do?**

Tammy: I've been going to a health salon. We do group exercise there. These include leg lifts and sit ups to firm the stomach, various body movements for the hips and running for the whole body. Some of the exercises stimulate body co-ordination almost like ballet.

Jim: I do two kinds of exercises: one type to build up muscle strength, and the other to build up circulation (lungs and blood flow). As a youth, I never got into playing sports. So I did very little to get my body into shape. I see now that was wrong. We are a whole being — a spirit, soul and body, and we need to exercise and discipline our whole being. For years, I misused my body and eventually it caught up with me and almost destroyed me. Fortunately, it was not too late and God has renewed my strength through exercise.

To build muscle tone, I work on doing sit ups and leg lifts. For my arms and chest, I lift weights regularly. Weights also help build the muscles in my legs and thighs. For improving circulation and lung power, jumping rope and swimming works best for me. These types of exercises, I feel, are most important because they build up the heart and reduce the stress on it.

This may sound surprising but I was never really taught what were the best exercises to develop the different muscle groups and slenderize the needed areas of my body. Therefore, it has really helped my exercise program to learn about this from Eric Orders — one of our PTL staff. We're including some of these suggested exercises for men and women in the Appendix. (See Appendix III.)

Jeff: **Did you find exercising difficult to get into and hard to keep at?**

Tammy: I had to commit myself to doing it. It helped that a friend started going with me. We could encourage one another to go — much like the AA idea. I never was real active in sports so I didn't have a natural desire to exercise. And I couldn't say I really enjoyed the exercising at first, but I could stand before a mirror and see the fat going and the body firming before my eyes. That was certainly encouraging.

Jim: Keeping at it is a lot harder than getting started. I started naturally with the physical demands on the world trip. I've had a positive incentive of better health that has kept me going since, but the time requirements of my daily routine often tempt me to crowd it out of my schedule.

So many people think of exercise as work. It doesn't have to be. I don't particularly like running but there are exercises that I do enjoy. So I concentrate on them. There are enough different ways to exercise that everyone can find at least one they enjoy. It may require an investment of time and money, but it is better spent than on doctor bills and time in bed or in the hospital.

Jeff: **Was there a point when exercise got easier?**

Tammy: Yes, I remember trying to run a certain number of laps, I thought I would die. But I decided I was going to make it no matter what. Pretty soon I got a second wind and I felt just great, I didn't want to stop. For me, it has something to do with discipline. My fleshly nature no longer fights, as it did against exertion, so I can enjoy exercise much more now.

Jim: Exercising is easier now that my body is used to it and I've established a discipline. My strongest discipline is still to stay healthy. I've known what it is to be sick unto death. Mentally, it is a constant challenge to keep exercise a daily priority. I've often been tempted to think I can get by without it today. It's easy to get out of the habit and then hard to get back into the discipline again.

Jeff: **How long do you exercise and how often?**

Tammy: Many people think you have to exercise for hours to do any good. But in just one hour of exercise class, three times a week, I can keep in shape. For my own enjoyment, I like to stay on the machines for another half hour each time I go.

Jim: I try to exercise anywhere from 30 minutes to an hour every day. Certain exercises like jumping rope for 5 to 10 minutes and doing some sit ups are so important that I do them daily. Some of the other exercises, like swimming, can be limited to 2 or 3 times a week. Time limitations should not hinder a person from physical exercise. New programs like the Air Force aerobics plan (See Appendix IV.) can show a person how to get good exercise in just 15 to 20 minutes a day. Ten minutes of strenuous jumping rope is equivalent to more than 30 minutes of jogging. Even 5 minutes a day would improve most people's health and well-being.

Once a person decides the value of exercise, it is amazing how easy it is to fit some daily exercise into one's lifestyle — deciding to take the stairs instead of the elevator, choosing to walk instead of taking the car on a short trip, ways to spend family time in physical activity, mowing your own lawn, etc.

Jeff: **How fast can you expect to see results?**

Tammy: That depends primarily on where you are when you start. In five months, I lost 24 pounds and 20 inches in measurements, including 6 inches off my hips and 4 inches off my waist. That may not sound like a lot but my dress size has dropped from 11 to 5 and slacks size from 12 to 8.

For most, this is the reward of exercising. The weight comes off faster. I could see the difference almost daily. I believe most people quit their diets, because they don't see results soon enough. Exercising can help these types of people see results sooner.

Jim: I think you should begin to feel healthier and have more vitality almost immediately if you take exercising seriously. If one is exercising primarily to lose weight, the desired results may take a little longer. I'm told a person has to run a mile to burn off 100 calories. The first month I did burn off quite a bit of fat and I could see it in the reduction of my waist size. I could also see my muscles toning up and firming within a couple of weeks.

Jeff: **What time of day do you exercise?**

Tammy: I exercise in the early afternoon because it's the

most convenient time. I think the time of day one exercises should be that time that best fits one's schedule. But it should be the same time all the time.

Jim: I exercise mainly in the morning. It stimulates my body and circulation — making me more alert. It also happens to be the best time I can fit it into my schedule.

If I am not bushed, I'll also do a few exercises before I fall into bed. That's a good tonic for restful sleep.

Jeff: **How about running?**

Tammy: I try to do some running a couple times a week. I think the amount of running one should do depends on the individual. Running is a good exercise in that it exercises most of the muscles and stimulates the lungs and blood circulation.

Jim: I have not done much running simply because I find it is hard to fit the necessary time in my schedule. Also, a Christian chiropractor whom I respect highly has expressed to me concern that daily running on a hard surface is rough on our body's frame, and can result in bone problems. I believe that theory just enough not to get convicted that I'm not running more.

There is something about long distance running (or swimming) that Tammy mentioned before which is so important. It taxes the body beyond its natural desires. We feel we can't go on, but when we say to our body, "Yes, you can; you must." we find we can. Then we've gained control over our self nature in that area. That is part of self-control which is one of the fruits of the Holy Spirit.

Many people have never reached their potential because they've never stretched themselves to see what they can do with God's help. When we do this physically, it builds confidence and faith in other areas of our life. Paul says, "when we are weak, then we are strong." He means that when we come to the place where our own strength is no more and we call on God's strength, we can walk in divine strength — in spirit, soul, and body. Our Lord condemned the Laodiceans because they were self satisfied. They didn't exert themselves physically or spiritually. Our Christian walk is a race; it requires great inner strength.

Jeff: **Do you eat before exercising?**

Tammy: Yes, we have a light lunch before we go to class. It doesn't upset the stomach and we feel better doing the exercise.

Jim: No, I eat breakfast after I exercise. After I exercise, my body relaxes and is ready for nourishment.

Doctor   It is not good to do heavy exercising after a big
Gyland: meal. The body needs to relax in order to digest
         the food we eat. We strain both our stomach and
         our heart when we exercise right after eating.

Jeff: **Tammy, you do your exercising in a group.
         Do you and Jim think that is important?**

Tammy: Very, very important. I don't see how people
         can do it alone. The fellowship, the encourage-
         ment, the commitment to being somewhere at a
         certain time are all positive influences to be
         faithful. I usually exercise with Christian
         girlfriends and we have fun and encourage one
         another.

Jim: I can see where group exercise can be a positive
         motivator and encouraging. I don't believe it is
         necessary, however. I exercise alone because it
         is not convenient to do otherwise.

         More important than exercising as a group, I
         think, is to do physical activities as a family. It can
         then be both healthy and enjoyable. Family
         sports like tennis or bowling or skating or skiing
         are great. Every family should do at least one
         regularly. Even getting out and walking together
         can do so much good — both physically and
         mentally.

         If you are not living with family, surround
         yourself with friends who are active and positive
         people. I find most gluttons stick together, paci-

fying each other — not realizing they are destroying one another in self deception.

Jeff: **You would then recommend going to a health salon?**

Tammy: Yes, I would, The fact that you're paying for the exercises is a positive stimulus. The accurate scales, the continual record keeping of your weight, the encouragement and admonishment from those in leadership and the expertise in telling which are the most effective exercises for the particular muscles you need to work on — all these are so important.

Jim: Going to a health spa could be a good thing, especially because of the facilities available. Many have those belt driven running machines where you can jog without fear of damaging your frame. The availability of different types of weights and machines can help you concentrate on certain muscles you may want to tone up. Indoor swimming pools and handball and squash courts are all helpful incentives in exercising.

Jeff: **Tammy, what if no health salon is accessible?**

Tammy: I would suggest you organize a small group of women in the neighborhood with similar interests. Establish regular meeting times for exercises. Get accurate scales and keep records.

Jeff: **Do the exercise machines help?**

Tammy: They help me to feel better, so I like them. Like anyone else, I have tension and that tension makes my body hurt, especially when I don't exercise. The exercise machines help me work off some of that tension, plus set up good circulation of the blood.

The machines cannot, like some might suggest, take off weight. You must get the body to do the work.

Jim: They are helpful in doing specific exercise to work on specific muscles. However, lack of machines, finances or facilities can be no excuse for not exercising. The three most important exercises in most all exercise programs require essentially no monetary investment or equipment. These are sit-ups, jumping rope and walking or running.

Jeff: **Should a person go to a doctor before dieting and exercise?**

Tammy: I think so. I didn't even know what weight I probably should be until I went to the doctor. Checking your height and frame can pretty well determine a person's proper weight. If a person has any physical problems whatever, a doctor's suggestions can be helpful in the amount and kinds of exercises that are best.

Jim: Definitely. Because of insurance coverage, I am
            required to take a physical every year, but I think
            that is good.

            Before one gets involved with anything
            strenuous like jogging, one should get a physical.
            A doctor can often give a person some good tips
            about their specific health needs in relation to diet
            and exercise.

Doctor   I certainly agree with Jim here. I think regular
Gyland: medical check-ups are a good idea and especial-
            ly important in people past age 40. A careful
            evaluation of the heart is especially important for
            those radically changing their exercise and
            dietary habits.

Jeff: **Can exercise be dangerous?**

Tammy: Not if one does it properly. That's where a doc-
            tor's advice and group exercise can help.

Jim: Doing too much at once can be dangerous. But
            that shouldn't be used as an excuse for not exer-
            cising. Both of my folks are in their seventies and
            they exercise daily. My dad still carries one of the
            highest averages in our PTL bowling league.

Jeff: **Dr. Gyland, are most medical doctors now**
            aware of the need for exercise and good
            nutrition and its healthful effects on the
            body?

Doctor
Gyland:
The current jogging and exercise craze has not elluded the medical profession, and I hope to some degree we have stimulated it. The science of nutrition is exploding to varying degrees in the medical profession. I would say it is the doctor's duty to advise the patient about nutrition and exercise. It is still the patient's responsibility to carry out the proper exercise and eating habits.

This is where nutrition knowledge is coming into focus. I believe that the day of junk foods is waning. I see where the public is rising up against the advertisement of sweets and sweetened cereals on children's TV programs. These are good indicators.

Jeff:
Has exercise made you feel healthier?

Tammy:
Physically, I haven't noticed much difference as I'm healthy and have always felt good — except now my knees, with which I've always had a problem, are stronger. Before I started exercising, I had to wear knee braces on my knees in the winter, because of the pain in them. This winter I haven't had to wear them and the pain has been much less. Mentally, I'm a lot healthier. I've begun to like the way I look and that gives me much more confidence.

Jim:
It has literally saved my life. Ten years ago when I was working for CBN and hosting the 700 Club, I let financial and emotional pressures get to me until I nearly had a nervous breakdown. I

became physically ill and my nerves were so jangled that I was falling apart inside.

Fortunately, God led me to a good doctor. Instead of stuffing me with pills, she correctly diagnosed my problem. She said, "You are getting no physical exercise. This is your problem. You need some physical outlets like sports or fishing to bring your life into balance." I tried her suggestion and it worked.

During that time I can remember a kid coming up to me while I was mowing the lawn. He asked me if he could mow it for me. I'm sure he didn't understand my reply when I said, "No thanks, I'm saving my life."

Everybody, young and old alike, needs an outlet that involves physical activity. It may be mowing the lawn, tending a garden, sports, bowling or fishing. A person should try to balance their mental and physical strain so they are equal or close to it.

Now that I am fit and healthy, exercise is still the great energizer of my day. It stimulates me for action and makes my mind and body alert. This is why I try to exercise regularly in the morning.

During the night, my body's digestive system has taken the protein and nutrients of the food I've eaten and converted them into amino acids and sugars (stored energy). When I exercise, I get this stored energy into "action," feeding the cells from my brain on down, so I feel alert, but if I don't exercise and eat, the body is simply forced to store up more food without being really activated and as a result, I feel tired and listless, and drag through the day.

This is the whole idea behind "pep" pills. They artifically send chemicals into the blood stream that activate this stored up energy. However, they are psychologically addictive and are harmful to the body. Exercise is far more effective and has no harmful side effects to the body.

Jeff: **Do you now sleep better?**

Tammy: Maybe, a little, I've never had a problem sleeping except when I was under great emotional stress. Exercise has helped several of my friends to sleep better.

Jim: Exercise has definitely improved my sleeping habits. One of the most important things about exercise is that it builds up the heart to allow it to work harder and improves the circulation of the blood. With exercise the heart can work harder and beat slower, which keeps the body more relaxed, so sleep comes easier. I now sleep great. As a result I wake up more refreshed and zealous to take on another day.

Good sleep is also a spiritual matter. God says we are to "rest in the Lord." When we get self under control in the areas of diet and exercise, we are no longer driven by hunger and tiredness. Then we experience peace and rest. We can really rest — rest in the Lord — not driven by hunger (Psalm 37).

A good way to check whether you are overly tense is to check your hands when you are sitting in church or just watching TV. If they are balled up in a fist, likely you are too tense and need to relieve that stress.

Jeff: **How about your spiritual health?**

Tammy: Hasn't affected it at all.

Jim: Physical and spiritual health are interrelated. I have already shared that. I went through a period of severe emotional strain that had to do with the fact that I had no physical outlet and had poor eating habits. I have counselled many people with depression whose main problem was they let their body get out of shape and they were eating all kinds of poisons. They were killing their bodies — no wonder they felt bad! Depression can also be a warning signal of allergic reactions to food or chemical additives.

As I have travelled, some of the people that are in the worst physical shape were Christians. This should not be the case. History tells us that in the early church there were groups of heretics called "gnostics" who felt that the only thing that was important was spiritual knowledge and experience. They felt that anything material or of the body was evil. I've met some people that bordered on that philosophy today.

They think the only thing of value is the Spirit and every thing else is carnal. But when we offer ourselves to God, we offer spirit, soul and body that He may sanctify and redeem them all for His purpose.

Jeff: **Tammy, isn't there a danger that through exercise you'll become muscle bound and lose your femininity?**

Tammy: Just the opposite. Exercise and dieting has really helped me feel feminine again. I had gotten so chubby that my tummy stuck out as far as my breasts. I was embarrassed to walk across the bedroom. I couldn't wear nice scimpy and frilly lingerie, because of my bulges. I looked terrible in a swimming suit. Jim says I'm now a new woman. As for developing bulging muscles, that is one advantage of exercising at a health salon. They can show you what exercises to do, and how much, to prevent that from happening. For the first time in years my bust and hip measurements are the same. My tummy is flat and my waist is small again.

Jeff: **But doesn't exercising increase your appetite?**

Tammy: No. This is a popular misconception. It actually decreases my appetite. I don't want to eat after exercising. I think this is because the exercising increases my circulation and therefore properly nourishes the body.

Jim: Tammy is right, exercise actually reduces my appetite. Part of it is the fact that I'm learning to bring my body under control, and that includes food intake. The body is a wonderful creation of God. It has a way of telling us what it needs. When we exercise and tune our body properly, it creates in us desires for fruits, protein and vegetables — the good foods.

Jeff: **Then you have been eating less since you have gotten on your diet and exercise program?**

Tammy: Yes, I used to live to eat, I now eat to live. I was both a "coke-aholic" and a "sweetaholic." I loved pastry and junk food. When we used to go to McDonalds, I would have a large burger, french fries, Coke and vanilla shake. I might then top that off with a hot fudge sundae. Now if we go, I eat a ¼ pound hamburger with the top bun off and drink a vanilla milkshake and I'm full.

Jim: Exercise makes me feel better physically and makes me alert and desirous of foods that are healthy to me. This attitude has helped me cut out junk foods and protect me from being tempted to stuff myself with food at a meal.

Just like a well run machine, if you put junk into your body, it will run like junk. But if you properly care for it, the body will run properly.

Jeff: **Did you have to starve yourself to cut down like that?**

Tammy: No, starving never works over the long haul. A person must have a balanced diet and if you cut out a lot of food and starve yourself, your body is going to react strongly. For me it was better to cut down gradually. I found that I didn't need all the food I was eating. I discovered that I didn't always need to eat everything on my plate to get full. I could leave some of it. For example, on Thanksgiving, I decided to splurge. I put on my plate turkey, dressing, potatoes, gravy, rolls, baked beans, vegetables and dessert. I was filled before I ate half of it. Instead of stuffing myself like before, I just left it on the plate.

Jim: I've done pretty much as Tammy. Mainly, it has been cutting down the quantity of my food intake. I only eat enough to satisfy me physically. God's word has helped in this. Proverbs 13:25 says "The righteous eateth to the satisfying of his soul: but the belly of the wicked shall want." I used to think I had to always finish everything on the plate (Boy Scout philosophy); God helps me to know how much is satisfying and leave the rest.

What I've tried to cut out of my diet is sweets and heavy starches. Like Tammy, I had built up quite a desire for sweets, desserts and junk foods. My around the world trip experience was like going "cold turkey." I don't recommend that for everyone. However, seeing the world's hunger would be an enlightening experience for most Americans. Remember Tammy's and my previous experience in trying to cut off sweets: "cold turkey didn't work." There is a good booklet, *The Junk Food Withdrawal Manual*[1], which is a very practical guide to better eating habits.

Since getting away from large quantities of sweets, I don't find myself hungering for these as much. I still slip occasionally with a dessert or sweets, but it doesn't make me give up.

A person dieting faces the same temptation as a Christian waging war against sin. A person is tempted with the line, "Just once won't do any harm." Then after the sinful act is done and judgment doesn't come immediately, one is tempted to think that he can get away with continuing the wrong thing. Then when a person continues in wrong he gets into trouble; Satan comes up and says, "You've really blown it now, you may as well give up."

[1] *The Junk Food Withdrawal Manual* by Monte Kline, Harvest Press, Fort Worth, TX 76105 (39 Cents).

When a person fails whether in sin or dieting, he or she should go to God immediately to ask for forgiveness and strength. In that way, no harm will be done. Everyone that is attempting to diet will sometimes stray, but the key is getting back on it right away. Discipline is important.

Doctor Gyland: Actually, starving yourself or fasting is not a bad way to diet. I found I can live happily and healthily on one meal a day. I don't like to do that regularly but with my busy lifestyle, it often happens. Certainly, not everyone can live on one meal a day. It depends on a person's metabolism. Some people, if they eat less, will want less food when they eat. Others, if they miss a meal, will get so hungry they will stuff themselves on the next day; so it is no advantage for them to cut down the number of meals they eat.

Jeff: **Have you had to cut out many foods from your diet?**

Tammy: Not really, I love sweets, ice cream and desserts and I haven't cut them out altogether. I still get ice cream or pie but I restrict myself to eat half of it. I've tried diets that cut out starches or this or that. It doesn't work for me over the long haul. I've learned that diets which totally cut out carbohydrates are unhealthy. The body needs some carbohydrates to convert into glucose to feed the brain.

Jim: I have developed a philosophy that is personal
          but it works for me. I ask, "If God didn't make this
          as food, does He really intend for me to eat it?" I
          even take that one step further to go back to the
          Old Testament law and try to eliminate from my
          diet those foods that God called unclean.

          I don't make it a strict law, but I do believe
          healthwise, it is best. I know the vision God gave
          Peter in Acts about the unclean animals, though I
          believe that God was speaking about an attitude
          in Peter, mainly about the Gentiles, and not, in
          fact, changing His views about what were the
          best foods for us to eat.

          I believe that God made all the animals for a pur-
          pose but not necessarily all for food for us. God
          created some as garbage collectors and I would
          put pigs in that category. Therefore, you can not
          force me to eat bacon and I will not eat an ex-
          cessive amount of pork. The high amount of
          grease and fat it contains is certainly not good for
          my health. I also try to limit my intake of shellfish
          meats. They require a lot of energy to burn off
          and so can be hard on the body.

Doctor   The most dangerous foods that Americans are
Gyland: regularly eating are those high in refined car-
          bohydrates and those high in animal fats. I agree
          totally with Jim that the guidelines about diet
          which God laid out in the Old Testament are for
          our good. Pork is perhaps the highest in fat con-
          tent among all the meats. Even "lean ham" is fill-

ed with fat. Beef also has a lot of fat content. I would suggest that people eat beef no more than 2 or 3 times a week. Fish and poultry are much better in providing protein without fat. The fat is very difficult to break down in the body and will eventually increase the load on the heart and produce hardening of the arteries. The animal or milk fat found in milk, cream or ice-cream, is certainly as hazardous to the health as the fat found in the pork. This dairy product source of fat is one which is frequently overlooked. However, in skim milk, yogurt, or cottage cheese, this fat has been removed.

Jeff: **Jim and Tammy, what does your diet consist of now?**

Tammy: My diet is basically what it used to be, but only eating half as much and cutting out as much sugar as possible. I like a wide variety of foods so I don't just cook and eat diet foods. Some of the foods we eat contain some refined starches and sugar, but I keep the amount small and make sure all the foods we eat are nutritious in some way.

Jim: My parents always believed in a balanced diet of meat, vegetables, fruit and potatoes. I still believe in that basic diet with slight alterations.

First, I fill my diet with whole grains — in cereals for breakfast and in any bread I eat. The white bread with its refined flour that we are used to eating is practically worthless to the body. You can take a slice of white bread and ball it up in your hand and see that it adds no fiber to the body. The joke goes, "the bugs don't get in the flour anymore because there is not enough nutrition to keep them alive." There is some truth in that. The only bread I eat now is made from whole grains. (See Appendix V for recipe.) It is the same bread we feed our guests and Partners that visit PTL.

Vegetables, fresh if possible, make up a large part of my diet. To retain their nutrients, they should be cooked as little as possible. Steam cooking is a good way to keep the nutrients in vegetables. I also eat salad regularly along with vinegar and unsaturated oil (olive) dressing.

At every meal, I will have fruit in some form, either whole or juice. Fresh fruit is best but canned fruit or juice is fine as long as it doesn't contain the heavy sweet syrup in which most fruit is canned. We usually get our canned fruit out of the dietectic section. If a person regularly adds fruit and fiber to their diet, they will never have to worry about elimination problems.

Because of the harmful fat content I don't eat as much meat as I once did, and I see that the meat I do eat is lean. I usually eat a starch, like potatoes or rice, one meal a day. A baked potato is not harmful to my diet as long as I don't put a lot of butter or sour cream on it. (See Appendix VI for sample diet plan.)

Just by eating good foods and cutting out the junk foods, I have lost 24 pounds. I guarantee that if a person is overweight, he or she will automatically lose weight just by eating good foods. A simple diet for anyone to follow is to replace their sugar and sweets with fruits and fruit juices; replace their heavy starches and refined flour products with whole grains and reduce their animal fat intake.

Jeff: **You all entertain a lot. How do you entertain and still diet?**

Tammy: For Jim and me, recreation and entertainment has always centered around eating — whether it is having people over or going out to restaurants. We still do this only we've changed our eating habits some. Instead of going to maybe like an Italian or German restaurant with real rich food, we'll go to a Chinese restaurant now. We've found we enjoy it and it is much less fattening. When we have people over, the only difference is that we eat less and the desserts I make will likely not be as rich.

Jim: Actually, I find it easier to keep on my diet in a restaurant rather than eating at home. Eating out, I can choose what is best for me to eat and order that. If you find you have trouble staying on a diet while eating out, it may be because you are not disciplining yourself in your diet. For some people, it is harder for them to stay on a diet while entertaining others. But it is important "not to throw out the baby with the bath water." Sharing food together has always had an important place in scripture — from Abraham preparing a meal for the angel of the Lord, to our Lord cooking breakfast for the disciples after His resurrection. Jesus said "I stand at the door and knock; If any man hear my voice and open the door, I will come in and sup with him." Sharing meals together is a wonderful means of Christian fellowship.

One of the most pleasant memories of my childhood was going to Grandma Irwin's house. She always had something delicious to eat. I will be eternally grateful for her hospitality.

Doctor Gyland: Regarding eating in a restaurant, I believe people should be concerned with what they order. The deep fried foods can be very high in fat content and unhealthy. Beware of meats camouflaged by breading and rich sauces. Order individually cut meat and know what you're getting. Jim and Tammy's suggestion of Oriental food is good. Most of that type of food is nourishing, and low in refined carbohydrates and harmful animal fat.

Jeff: **How about desserts?**

Tammy: I love desserts and I think most people do too. But I have found that the desserts I now like aren't real bad for my diet in small amounts. Naturally sweetened desserts like fruit satisfy that craving for something sweet but don't have a lot of calories. There are a number of desserts that are light and fruity. I enjoy ice cream and so I will have some occassionally. But these new yogurt bars with only 60 calories are almost as good.

Jim: I try not to eat desserts. If something really appeals to me, I'll eat one or two bites of it. This is enough to satisfy my taste for it. It is the large amount of sugar in most desserts that is unhealthy. The average American eats a whopping 150 pounds of sugar every year.

It was actually Dr. Gyland here who on PTL about a year ago brought to my attention the great hazards of refined sugars to the body. He can explain the why and wherefores. I just know that since eliminating refined sugars from my diet, I am stronger and healthier. And to do the things that God has called me to, I need all the strength I can muster.

Doctor Gyland: I grew up in good Southern tradition with a regular heavy diet of desserts in our family. For many years, my father suffered unknowingly with hypoglycemia (low blood sugar). So, much like Tammy, I became a sweetaholic. Since then, I've learned that sweets are physically addictive. They put a person into a vicious cycle of food frustration. Within minutes of eating something with high sugar content, the sugar gets into the bloodstream and causes the blood sugar level to rise. This causes the pancreas to produce insulin.

The insulin enables the liver and muscles to withdraw the sugar from the blood and store it as starch or else change it into fat.

Now some sugar is fine to provide energy for the body, but when the body gets a flood of sugar from something like a rich dessert, it causes the pancreas to produce too much insulin which causes the liver to withdraw too much sugar from the blood. So the result is low blood sugar and feeling tired. The person feels the need then for more sugar and most of the sugar taken in becomes stored as fat rather than used as energy for the body.

When I was an Air Force Flight Surgeon I had a man come to my office who was grossly overweight and was feeling continually tired. When I asked him what he did when he was feel-ing that way, he said he would eat a candy bar and that would help for a little while.

When I showed him the vicious cycle he was in and suggested to him a high protein diet that cut out most sweets, he immediately lost 45 pounds and regained his normal strength.

For some people it is easier to do as Jim and Tammy did and cut down on sweets and use sweet substitutes when ever possible. For others to leave off sweets totally so changes the desires of the palate that they are very happy to do without sweets. After their body gets reeducated, they actually find sweet desserts and sweet beverages distasteful.

Substitutes for sweet desserts include yogurt, the unsweetened kind, cottage cheese, fresh fruits or nuts.

Jeff: **Dr. Gyland, do many people in America suffer with hypoglycemia?**

Doctor Because of its incidence in my own family, Func-
Gyland: tional Hypoglycemia has been a major field of personal interest to me. And I've discovered that tens of thousands of Americans suffer with this disease — many of them, unknowingly. Besides its toll on body energy and strength, for some, it is the first step toward the worse disease of diabetes.

The incidence of hypoglycemia has been underestimated by the medical profession for quite a few years, but it has now become so well recognized that the House of Delegates of the Florida Medical Association unanimously voted to ask the State Legislature to require a blood sugar test as well as an alcohol test on anyone suspected of drunken driving, since low blood sugar causes people to act as if they are intoxicated.

Symptoms of hypoglycemia may include anxiety, fear, phobias, nervousness, fainting spells, even convulsions at times, mental confusion, irritability, and breaking out in cold sweats. There is a fairly simple test which people can take themselves to check whether or not they might be suffering from this disease. (See Appendix VII for this self check test.) If a person's results from this test is positive, one should consult a doctor for further testing.

Jeff: **What about snacks?**

Tammy: I was horrible about eating snacks and junk food. When we would go to a movie, I had to have a candy bar, a cold drink, a box of candy coated almonds and buttered popcorn. I've not been able to go without snacks altogether but instead of eating junk foods, I now eat either an apple, sunflower seeds or plain popcorn. I think a lot of snacking for me is just wanting to put something in my mouth. Sunflower seeds and popcorn, because they're small, seem filling without content.

Jim: Snacking hits home on perhaps the greatest problem with our diet in America — and the problem is spiritual rather than physical. About ⅔ of Americans are overweight from overeating, yet we spend nearly 25% of our food dollars on snack food to supplement our already gluttonous diet. Our desire for snacks comes largely from a psychological conditioned response from our need of love. In childhood, food is given us in acts of love by parents. We come to identify in our minds the receiving of food with receiving love. When we reach for a snack, we may be saying, "I need love."

How often I have turned to the refrigerator or cupboard for a snack after a bad or frustrating day instead of turning to prayer. Recently, I had a guest on the PTL Club program who lost 200 pounds after she found Christ and realized she was loved by God. She had been looking for love in food and snacks.

Isaiah 58 tells us how to free ourselves from this conditioned response. Isaiah says in verses 6 and 7 that if we fast as God desires, we will begin to give out our food to others and this will break the yoke. Fulfillment comes not just in receiving love but in giving love. This is the growing process — learning to give. When we share love, we are fulfilled and are freed of the bondage of gluttony.

I am not putting all snacking in this category. I believe a certain amount of snacking is fine.

For snacks, I will eat either fruits, nut mix or popcorn. Unbuttered popcorn is perhaps the best for dieters. A handful of popcorn will give you a lot of bulk to eat and not many calories. It also adds roughage which the body needs. Nuts are also good in that they give the body needed protein.

Doctor Gyland: Have you ever heard of that potato chip commercial, "Bet you can't eat just one?" The ad is true. They are addictive because they are also mainly carbohydrates, just in a little different form. Much better snacks are those that have some nutritional value. The ones that Jim and Tammy mentioned are good. You may find health food bars or other items at the health food store appealing for snacks. You can create your own healthful foods more inexpensively by buying the ingredients from your local grocery store and making your own mixtures.

Jeff: **How about drinks?**

Tammy: I've always hated drinking just water and I still don't like water. When I was small, our family could only afford for us kids to have soft drinks once a year, on the Fourth of July. That was such a special treat that when I got to the point that I could afford Cokes, I got addicted to them. Once I lost over five pounds just by cutting out Cokes, but I could not go without drinks that were either fizzy or were sweet. So now I carry my own artificial sweeteners and drink unsweetened tea or diet drinks. Some diet drinks I like and others I don't.

Jim: I drink a lot of water. It is void of calories and healthy to the body. Water is necessary to purge the body of poisons we take in with our normal diet. I also endeavor to cut down my intake of coffee. The caffeine in the coffee speeds up the heart which isn't healthy. Instead I try to drink natural fruit juices. They contain the vitamins, minerals, and natural sweeteners that the body needs for energy without taxing the digestive system.

I would like to reiterate what Tammy said about soft drinks. When you read the label on the can, the first thing it says is sugar. That means it is the major ingredient in the product.

You can look at candy labels and see the same thing. Even products like batter coatings for meats are more than 50% sugar. We should read the labels of the products we buy and be aware of what we're getting. Most of us have depended on government standards to protect us from harmful ingredients. I believe we should show personal interest in ingredients.

If I must have a soft drink, I'll make sure its artifically sweetened. I think it is interesting that some reports trying to discredit artificial sweetners as hazardous to the body were funded by the sugar industry. And these reports have not been fully substantiated.

Doctor Gyland: It's almost hard to find drinks that are good for us. Finally, most vending machines now also offer diet drinks in their soft drink selection. Again, the main thing to watch here is the caffeine and sugar intake in the drinks. Caffeine is harmful even taken without sugar but most of the caffeine beverages also include a lot of refined sugar. I would recommend artificial sweeteners over refined sugar.

Jeff: **It sounds like dieting has become to you a way of life.**

Tammy: Definitely. I think that is one of the big secrets in successful dieting. I haven't gone on this diet with the idea that it will last three months or even a year. This is the way I'm going to eat for the rest of my life. Dieting is largely a battle within, not without.

Jim: Dieting must be a way of life. If a person is overweight, the weight just didn't happen to get there by accident. A person must realize that his or her old pattern of eating was unhealthy and turn from it to a better way. Like a decision for Christ, that should be a lifetime decision if it is to work and last. Dieting is no more a project than being a Christian is being good just during the season of Lent.

I believe that dieting success is 75% mental attitude. Most of the battle is within rather than without. Once a person is convinced of the truth in his or her mind (this is where knowing of the truth of the Bible in this area is vital), the devil can no longer get a foothold. Esau let the devil take his hunger out of control and it cost him his birthright. The devil would desire to do the same with people today.

Just as Esau later wept bitter tears to no avail for his mistake, there are many people that now wish they had exercised more and eaten better foods earlier in life.

The older a person gets, the more he or she appreciates good health. Many people would give a million dollars or more for good health. But it is not something you can buy back, you must work at it and discipline to get it.

Jeff: **Do you think that proper dieting is largely a learning process?**

Tammy: Yes. Every one of us is different. Each of our bodies are tuned differently and need different things to keep our bodies nourished. A dock worker is going to use up more energy than a file clerk, so he needs a different diet, and needs to discover what is right for him. A lot of it must be done by trial and error.

Jim: I agree that different people with different lifestyles and metabolisms may need different diets, so it becomes a learning process, but total body health is more discipline and applying good health sense than individual knowledge. Successful dieting requires commitment — not to a project but to a new way of life of eating good food.

Doctor Gyland: I believe that proper dieting is a learning process but it is largely a decision. Just like in the Christian life, many times it takes years for us to come to the place where we will receive Christ and His help. Many people don't think about proper dieting until long after they have established bad eating habits and reaped a miserable harvest.

Everyone has a different metabolism and it doesn't do any good to fret and get jealous of the people who can eat and eat and never get fat. Even the nutrition experts can't always figure out why this is so. If God hasn't blessed us in this way, we simply need to recognize that and decide what we are going to do to get back in good health.

God hasn't promised that He will always be easy, but He is just. All of us have different trials to face. If the other person is not tried in the area of dieting like we are, he or she will certainly face a trial in another area of life.

Jeff: **Do you eat breakfast?**

Tammy: I find I am busy in the morning. I'm not thinking about food so I don't get hungry. In this I relate to what the Bible says about the "not eating the bread of idleness." So I usually only have a glass of orange juice for breakfast. By lunch time, I'm real hungry and will eat a big meal then, unless I'm going to exercise class.

Jim: Breakfast is the foundation of my diet. I always eat a big breakfast. I will have juice and a large bowl of whole grain cereal (See Appendix V for recipe.) to add fiber to my diet. Then I'll always have a vegetable and some fruit, usually an apple and a banana. The potassium in bananas is healthy for the body. If I feel I want some protein I'll also eat an egg with a little steak occasionally.

Doctor   The importance of breakfast is dependent on a
Gyland: person's metabolism and energy needs. I would
recommend that a person whose job requires
stress and/or physical strength eat a good
breakfast. Active children should get a good
breakfast, also.

Active children should get a good breakfast even
more than adults because by mid-morning in
their classes if they get hungry it is not convenient
for them to eat until lunch time. Most adult jobs
these days have a provision for a mid-morning
type of snack break if it is needed.

What Jim is saying about the fiber is it is vital for
good health. Without any doubt fiber lowers the
cholesterol level of the blood and reduces the incidence of gall stones. Most medical experts
believe it reduces much of the cancer in the in-
testinal tract. It probably also reduces the incidence of appendicitis and heart disease.

Fiber provides the necessary roughage for the
body and keeps the wastes flowing through the
body. Without the fiber the intestines fill up with
gas and hard stool. This produces pressure and
irritation to these body organs. The foods highest
in fiber are the brans, cabbage and other green
vegetables. Lettuce unfortunately is a good filler
food but is mostly water and has very little fiber.

Jeff: **What about fasting?**

Tammy: Metabolisms are different and not everyone can fast. I am one of those who cannot fast in my own strength. If God were to speak to my heart about fasting for a particular need, I know He would give me the strength and grace to do it.

Jim: We've already talked about the spiritual side of fasting, of learning to give in order to free oneself of the bondage of receiving. Fasting is not only spiritually edifying but it is physically healthful. It is a good way to cleanse the body of built up toxins, to build new reserves of energy, and burn off unwanted weight.

I never used to be able to fast and work. I would get headaches and become very weak. What was happening was that my sugar intake was so high that when I didn't eat, it was like going through withdrawal. This happens to most people when they fast. Now that I've cut out most sugar, I can fast and work, even for several days, and still feel strong and alert.

Doctor   Fasting is one of the best ways to lose weight.
Gyland: Tammy is right: metabolisms are different and not everyone can fast. But most everyone can learn to fast and reap rich physical, mental and spiritual benefits out of doing so.

Medically, it is proven that most people who are not diabetic, can fast up to 40 days on just water and vitamins without harming the body. Now certainly a person shouldn't start with a forty day fast. Fasting for a couple of meals or one day is a good way to start.

The Orthodox Jews fasted one day a week. But interestingly, their day started at 6 PM, so they would have the evening meal early and the next evening have it late. In essence, they only skipped two meals.

Jeff: **Do you and Jim then eat different meals at home?**

Tammy: Sometimes. I try to cook a balanced meal at home. But if Jim wants something special for his diet, I'll also cook that.

For breakfast and lunch, it's everyone for himself usually.

Jeff: **Are you passing on your dieting and exercise discoveries to your children?**

Tammy: Definitely. Our children, like most, were heavy eaters of junk food and sugar filled drinks. Now that our diet has changed, we have fruit around the house and serve popcorn and snacks like the baked cheese balls made from corn meal. The kids' snacks have changed a great deal.

They still eat some candy and junk food and we don't prohibit it totally. We feel legalism here could cause a feeling of abnormality in the children. Beyond that, we just make sure they get balanced meals for their health.

We are also encouraging Tammy Sue in sports and exercise. We feel right now that is one of the most important ways we can teach her to learn about caring for her body.

Jim: Just expanding a little on what Tammy said, we want our children to grow up balanced and disciplined in spirit, mind, and body. We feel that some exercise and sports activity should be part of every young person's routine, so we emphasize sports and gym in our Heritage Academy school.

Tammy does serve the kids balanced meals, so they are balanced in that area.

Doctor   We are such creatures of habit and tradition that
Gyland: building good nutrition habits in our children is a must. And today it is so difficult.

It is especially important not to pressure little children to eat more than their bodies want them to eat. If a person learns this habit of eating just a little more than their body needs when they are a skinny five year old, then when they are a fat 40 year old they are apt to find difficulty in stopping the habit of cleaning their plate or eating a little more than their body wants. Also, sweets and desserts should not be a reward for cleaning their plates or for any other "good" behavior.

Our children are bombarded with advertisements of sweets on children's TV programs. When we go to the store or to a restaurant, someone is always shoving a "sucker" in our kids' faces. It's impolite and almost impossible to refuse to let the kids receive these handouts.

The best preventative I know is to provide good balanced meals and have nutritious snacks available rather than junk food. And it is impossible to teach our children if we don't have good eating habits ourselves.

Jeff: **Do you set goals in your dieting?**

Tammy: Yes. But I set realistic goals. From the time I started, I only sought to lose 5 pounds at a time. Setting hard to reach goals can be very discouraging — at least for me.

Now I just try to lose something each time I weigh in at exercise class — even if it is only a quarter of a pound.

Jim: I set guidelines more so than goals. I know what approximate weight I should be for my size and I'm determined to be at or near that weight. I rather set goals in my exercise program — both at consistency and in building certain muscle areas.

Just as Tammy said, goals that are set in dieting must be reachable and set in small increments of weight. A few calories less everyday will add up in the long run. Successful dieting requires patience and this is where setting short term goals help. Prayer is just as important.

As Christians, we can approach dieting as well as all areas of life from a position of victory. We can apply John 15:7 ("If ye abide in me, and my words abide in you, ye shall ask what ye will, and it shall be done unto you") in prayer for God's help in controlling our weight and gaining better health.

God clearly understands our problems and needs in this area. Remember Jesus fasted for 40 days and "hungered." So with His grace and mercy, He will help us.

Jeff: **Do you believe everyone can learn to control their weight?**

Tammy: There are people that have thyroid problems that really need medical attention. But most of us can. We can all discover what's best for our bodies, set rules for ourselves and live by them. I now "eat to live" instead of "live to eat."

Jim: Yes. I believe the difficulty with weight control is that it requires consistency. In our country, we get shocked and up in arms when a tragedy kills 100 people. But things like alcoholism and being over-weight which eventually take thousands of lives, we seem to ignore. Often, we don't see the cost until it's nearly too late.

Doctor Everyone can learn to control their weight. It
Gyland: may not be exactly where they want it or exactly
where the chart (See Appendix II.) says they
should be, but metabolisms are different and
weight control should not be the only priority in
proper dieting. Good health should always take
priority.

Jeff: **What about diet pills?**

Tammy: I would never take them myself. Diet pills mainly
take off water weight so you're not really taking
care of the problem which is fat. The only way to
get fat off for good is to work it off and keep from
putting it back on by eating the proper foods.
Doctors tell me that it is bad for your body to take
off weight and put it back on numerous times. It
is actually better to stay 5 or 10 pounds
overweight than to keep fluctuating, so I don't
recommend these "quick-loss" diets.

Jim: I question the lasting value of all chemical diet
plans and project diets. I have never taken diet
pills but the experience of my co-host Henry
Harrison tells me to beware, especially of those
containing amphetamines. Henry has always
had a weight problem and about 15 years ago, a
doctor prescribed diet pills to control his weight.
It helped control his weight for a while but it caused him so much emotional trauma that even the
simplest decision caused a mental crisis. For
Henry it was supposed to be a short cut, but it
surely didn't get him to his desired end of good

health. As we shared before, the stimulation the body needs can naturally and safely be brought about by exercise.

Doctor Gyland: What Jim is saying is so true. No chemical pill is going to provide a shortcut to good health. In fact the majority of reputable doctors no longer use diet pills at all. If a person has a physical problem that prohibits weight control, he should see a doctor. But for most of us, pill and gimmick diet plans are not the answer. We need to make proper nutrition a way of life. Choose a diet we can live by and stick to it.

Jeff: **What about vitamins?**

Tammy: I never used to take them. I have a hard time swallowing them. As I don't like water, they are hard to take with Tab tickling your nose with its bubbles. But Jim has convinced me to start taking calcium and vitamin C. I haven't noticed any difference in how I feel, but I am sure they must be doing me some good. Maybe being faithful in taking vitamins shows up in rewards when you get older.

Jim: Vitamins have been vital to my health. During that period of severe emotional strain my body got really worn down. I was continually exhausted and would get dizzy without any physical exertion.

Vitamins really helped to build up my body and restore my strength. I especially recommend Vitamin C. It is a building vitamin and one the body doesn't store, so we need it often. Anytime I get an infection in my body, I take plenty of Vitamin C. It helps fight infections.

Because I am faced with stress in my day. I also take a complete B complex vitamin. I also take Vitamin E and supplement my mineral intake.

Lecithin is another important ingredient to the body which we often don't get enough of in our normal diet. This substance breaks down and dissolves hard fat cells and cholesterol, which causes hardening of the arteries.

Doctor Gyland: I can really appreciate Jim's benefits from vitamins in recovering from body and emotional collapse. However our modern food industry with quick freezing techniques and rapid transportation has resulted in good preservation of vitamins in our natural foods. So most medical authorities feel there is no reason for healthy Americans to take vitamin supplements over the age of two except during pregnancy and certain disease conditions. Of course, natural vitamins are essentially no different from synthetic vitamins.

It is interesting that in America well over *four billion dollars* are wasted each year by people taking mostly unneeded vitamins. It staggers the imagination to think how useful this four billion dollars a year would be in spreading the gospel of Jesus Christ by television such as PTL, instead of being excreted in the urine of people who didn't really need the vitamins in the first place.

Jeff: **What about natural foods?**

Tammy: I don't worry about natural or synthetic. I try to eat a balanced diet. I don't like honey or brans so I don't get into that.

Jim: I'm not a health food addict, but I believe strongly in natural foods for a healthy balanced diet. The whole grains and brans are needed for roughage. The fruits and vegetables are nutritious and strength building. Highly cooked and highly processed foods have lost all their nutritional value so I try to stay clear of them. Many of the chemicals added to lengthen their shelf life are not good for the body. When I eat bread, I make sure it is made from unrefined flour. And if something must be sweetened, I certainly won't use refined sugar. So I'll use honey or artifical sweeteners. The refinements of sugar and flour do destroy nutritional value.

Doctor   Food in its natural form is generally more
Gyland: nutritious. However, in the case of honey there is very little difference in the nutrition of natural honey and the refined cane sugar. Both are vir- tually pure sugar; one has been manufactured by man and the other by the honey bee.

Natural foods are certainly not mankind's salvation. Some chemical additives such as ascorbic acid and propionic acid are really natural compounds and we certainly don't want to "throw the baby out with the bath water" as Jim used the expression. Forty years ago there was much food poisoning from spoiled food and perhaps this was even one of the causes of the much more prevalent stomach cancer that we saw forty years ago then we see today in spite of the chemical additives. Therefore since modern food processing has virtually eliminated stomach cancer and food poisoning, it is not altogether bad.

Jeff: **How important is routine?**

Tammy: Very. Jim and I are very busy and have a lot of demands on our lives, so establishing routine is not easy. But it is vital in dieting. It has a lot to do with mental attitude. Once you decide to do something and establish a routine, there is little room for temptation and faltering. You've already committed yourself. Also, we are creatures of habit. So good eating habits are vital!

Jim: Routine is important in the sense that you decide you are going to do this or live this way, and you do it. It establishes your right decision, but routine should not be the law, but rather faith in God's direction.

Doctor   Routine is important in all areas of life — to
Gyland: reduce stress, to establish good patterns and to
          free us to do God's will. Once a person
          establishes a certain exercise pattern, he doesn't
          have to redecide every day whether or not he
          will or won't do this particular exercise; it just
          becomes a habit and leaves his decision making
          process free to tackle other decisions. The same
          is true of desserts and dieting in general. I know
          that having resolved not to eat desserts, I just
          form a habit of not eating desserts and the ques-
          tion just doesn't come to mind and I just don't eat
          them.

Jeff: **Is weighing important?**

Tammy: For me it is. It, too, has to do with mental at-
          titude, seeing the progress I've made. It is impor-
          tant to have good scales and to weigh at the same
          time of day each time.

          I used to weigh at the start of each exercise class
          — three times a week. Now that I am down to
          my proper weight, I weigh every day. If I see that
          I have gained a pound or so, I'll get tighter on my
          diet because it's much easier to lose one pound
          than five or ten.

Jim: If one is serious about dieting and weight control,
          regular and accurate weighing is vital. We
          wouldn't think of driving our car without a
          speedometer to measure our speed. I wouldn't
          consider doing the daily television program

unless I had an accurate clock which told me when to begin and finish.

Accurate weighing is the best and most accurate way of measuring progress in your diet. That means weighing the same time every day; I suggest in the morning when one gets out of bed. I also suggest weighing in the nude so you know exactly where you are in weight and you don't con yourself, estimating the weight of the clothes.

If goals in dieting are to mean anything, one must have accurate means of measuring ones' progress. Now that I'm down to my best weight, weighing helps me to maintain it and know when and if I can splurge occasionally.

Jeff: **Do you count calories?**

Tammy: No, I don't think that is practical in the long run. More so, I consider the portion size of what I eat to make sure I am not overdoing it. For example, my limit is now 2 pieces of pizza at most.

Jim: No, I consider the value and nature of what I eat more than the calorie values.

Doctor Gyland: I think most people should get a calorie counter book and check out the numbers of both calories and carbohydrates of the foods that they eat. They will be amazed at the number of calories and carbohydrates they are eating, and they will be encouraged to know how much they can improve their diet just by making little changes in their food intake.

The Hunter's book, "God's Answer to Fat" is the best I've seen so far on this subject. Once you have a good idea of what calories each food contains you should not find it necessary to count calories each meal.

Jeff: **What keeps you going on your diet in the face of temptation?**

Tammy: Mostly, I like what's happening to me, so I don't want to quit. People's compliments have been very encouraging. This may sound silly, but I suggest that women wear tight clothes or a girdle when eating. When they do, they feel filled up sooner and are less likely to overeat. Another protection against temptation and failure is knowing that I can keep to my diet. Therefore, to break it is a willful act.

Jim: What helps me is the conclusion that I reached in my own heart that gluttony for me is a sin. I've found with God's help, I can control my weight and food intake. So for me to willingly fall back into the trap of overeating or eating junk food is a sin.

Again, it is like Israel allowing their thoughts to slip back to the "goodies" of Egypt rather than looking to the Promised Land. The best way to overcome temptation is guard our thoughts, keeping them on good things and serving God and our fellow man.

This is not to say that there is no place for a big meal or feast. In the book of Nehemiah, when the Temple was rebuilt and the Book of the Law was read, Nehemiah called the people to a time of feasting, where they were to "eat the fat, and drink the sweet."

But the feast should be the special event, not the ordinary. And right after that, one should get right back to their regular routine.

Jeff: **Do you ever get discouraged?**

Tammy: Sure. At first, I was losing weight steadily. Then I hit a leveling off point where I didn't lose anything for 2 weeks. I almost gave up. But when I stuck it out, gradually I began to lose weight again. Women ought to be especially aware of body fluctuations with more fluids at certain times of the month and therefore not get discouraged during the times.

Jim: I get a little discouraged when I let the pressures of the day affect what I know I should be doing. When I let the pressures force out my scheduled exercise and when I don't take the time to eat right, I know I've blown it, and haven't really honored God with the right care of His vessel.

But I don't dwell on my discouragements. I know that nothing can separate me from God and His help, so I simply repent and re-commit myself to Him and His ways.

Jeff: **Has dieting and exercise affected your self image?**

Tammy: Definitely. I now begin to like the way I look and that gives me more confidence in every area of my life. More important, I've discovered that I can discipline myself and be faithful to a purpose, not just dieting and exercise, but whatever God calls me to do.

Jim: Yes. One of the greatest blessings is seeing my waist "shrink" three sizes. Now that I'm a size 29 x 30, I can easily buy precuffed pants off the rack. For the first time in over twenty years, my waist size is the exact same as it was when I was sixteen. I feel stronger and more confident. I'm developing physical strengths and disciplines I didn't know were possible for me. That is encouraging and stimulating for me.

Dieting and self-image work both ways. Valerie Issacs, the PTL guest that lost 200 pounds, told me she began to diet effectively when God changed her self-image and showed her she was a worthwhile person.

Jeff: **What do you think about each other's dieting and exercising?**

Tammy: I think it's great what Jim is doing. He has much more energy and looks better. But mostly I like it because it causes him to be happier with himself.

Jim: I have a new girl. I love it. We both feel happier and healthier.

Jeff: **What if one's husband or wife doesn't want the other at their best weight?**

Tammy: I feel that if a marriage partner tries to get the other to be at a weight that is not best for their health, he or she does not have the other person's interest at heart.

Jim: This often happens out of jealousy or competition. It is sad when couples vie with each other for the "top dog" position. True love always wants the best for the other person.

But it is very difficult, if not impossible, for a person to diet without the encouragement and cooperation of his or her mate. If a wife won't cook the right foods, how can the husband eat the right things? If the husband doesn't allow the wife sufficient grocery money for good and nutritious foods, the family's diet will suffer.

Doctor Finding a person that is not encouraging to
Gyland: his/her mate's efforts to good dieting or exercise is unusual. I suggest that couples decide together to diet and/or exercise just as Jim and Tammy have done. They will find the encouragement

and admonishments of each other very helpful, but remember, comments should be bathed in love and grace. God bless you as you step out in adventures to good health.

In conclusion, may I suggest I Corinthians 9:25, 27, "Every man that striveth for the mastery is temperate in all things. Now they do it to obtain a corruptible crown; but we an incorruptible. But I keep under my body and bring it into subjection; lest that by any means, when I have preached to others, I myself should be a castaway."

SUMMARY

Jim's ten most important steps to effective weight control.

1. Commitment — Determine to make a lifestyle of proper weight loss and maintenance.
2. Exercise your body daily.
3. Weigh yourself at the same time every morning. (Set short term goals and keep them.)
4. Read the labels of all the food you purchase. Know what you are eating.
5. Eat a nutritious breakfast of whole grain cereal, fruit, juices and vegetables.
6. For the first two months, cut out all soft drinks, white bread and all desserts from your diet.
7. Eliminate deep fried foods from diet.

8. Take time to eat nutritious meals (cut down trips to fast food chains).
9. Cut out pork and high animal fat meats.
10. Don't eat more than your body needs.

Tammy's ten most important steps to effective weight loss.

1. Exercise the entire body three times a week.
2. Stay away from junk foods — candy, cake, soft drinks, and fried potatoes.
3. Limit snacks to fruit, nuts, seeds, popcorn and unsweetened soft drinks.
4. Reduce food intake — try eating only half of what you put on your plate (or take half-portions).
5. If you must eat some sweets, eat something nutritious like a piece of a fruit pie or angel food cake.
6. When down to normal weight, weigh every morning.
7. When you gain a pound, reduce food intake that day. Easier to lose one pound than five.
8. When weight is lost, take clothes in for better appearance and recognition if clothes get tight again.
9. Establish proper mental attitude that you are not on a diet but on a new lifestyle pattern.
10. No matter how tired or disinterested, don't quit exercising even after you've lost weight. It is necessary for health and body firmness.

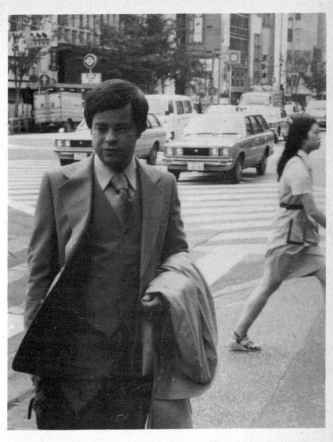

Jim's worldwide mission trip meant miles of walking daily. The hectic, exhausting pace was nonetheless physically exhilarating.

Phil Egert/Photographer

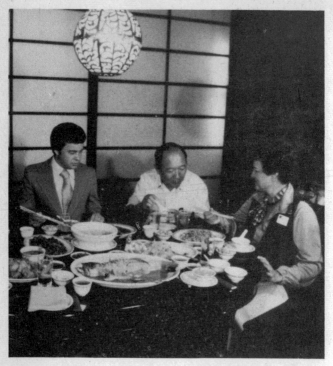

Oriental food of fish, poultry, steamed vegetables, nuts and rice, like this which Jim enjoyed on his world trip, is very nutritious and non-fattening.

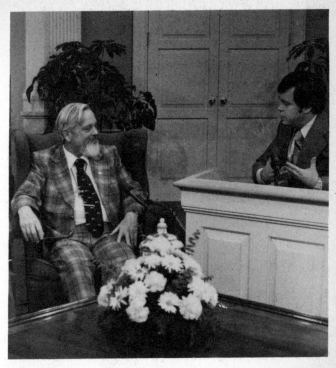

Dr. Stephen Gyland shares with Jim on the PTL Club the crippling impact of hypoglycemia, from which thousands of Americans suffer unknowingly.

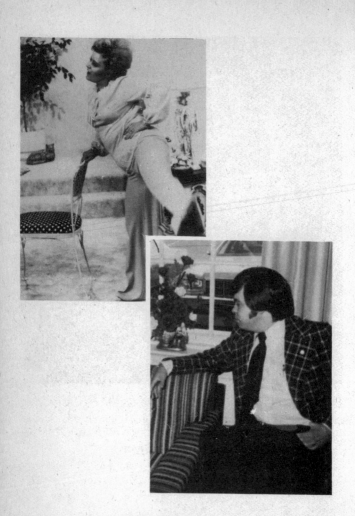

Jim and Tammy had a much "fuller" look before they went on their diets. Top: Tammy tries some exercises on the Tammy Faye show set. Bottom: Jim relaxes at his old office on Independence Blvd.

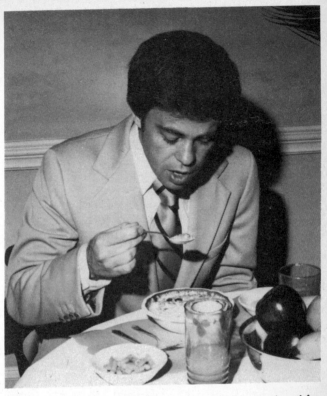

*The foundation of Jim's diet is a good, nutritious breakfast
with whole grain cereal, fruits and juices.*

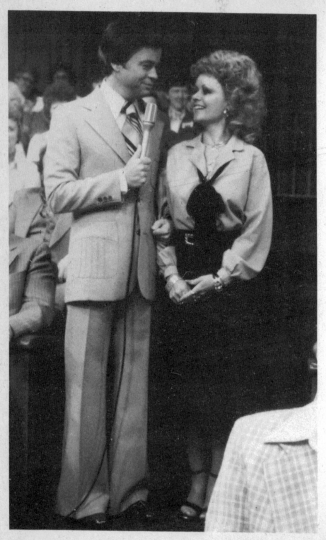

Jim & Tammy with their new looks on the daily PTL Club.

APPENDIX I
GOD'S PROMISES TO DIETERS

Satisfying the appetite of your soul —

I have esteemed the words of his mouth more than my necessary food.

—Job 23:12

How sweet are thy words unto my taste! Yea, sweeter than honey to my mouth!

—Psalms 119:103

Man shall not live by bread alone, but by every word that proceedeth out of the mouth of God.

—Matthew 4:4

But he said unto them, I have meat to eat that ye know not of.

—John 4:32

And Jesus said unto them, I am the bread of life: he that cometh to me shall never hunger; and he that believeth on me shall never thirst.

—John 6:35

For the kingdom of God is not meat and drink; but righteousness, and peace, and joy in the Holy Ghost.

—Romans 14:17

Fasting and physical strength —

And he arose, and did eat and drink, and went in the strength of the meat forty days and forty nights unto Horeb the mount of God.

—I King 19:8

Is not this the fast that I have chosen? to loose the bands of wickedness to undo the heavy burdens, and to let the oppressed go free, and that ye break every yoke? Is it not to deal thy bread to the hungry, and that thou bring the poor that are cast out to thy house?

—Isaiah 58:6, 7

Conquering overeating—

The righteous eateth to the satisfying of his soul; but the belly of the wicked shall want.

—Proverbs 13:25

Hast thou found honey? Eat so much as is sufficient for thee, lest thou be filled therewith, and vomit it.

—Proverbs 25:16

The full soul loatheth a honeycomb, but to the hungry soul every bitter thing is sweet.

—Proverbs 27:7

Eating Good Food—

Who satisfieth thy mouth with good things; so that thy youth is renewed like the eagles.

—Psalms 103:5

Prove thy servants, I beseech thee, ten days, and let them give us pulse (vegetables) to eat and water to drink.

—Daniel 1:12

Receiving God's help in your diet—

Trust in the Lord, and do good; so shalt thou dwell in the land, and verily thou shalt be fed. Delight thyself also in the Lord; and he shall give thee the desires of thine heart. Commit thy way unto the Lord; trust also in him; and he shall bring it to pass.

—Psalms 37:3-5

For verily I say unto you, That whosoever shall say unto this mountain, Be thou removed, and be thou cast into the sea; and shall not doubt in his heart, but shall believe that those things which he saith shall come to pass; he shall have whatsoever he saith. Therefore I say unto you, What things soever ye desire, when ye pray, believe that ye receive them, and ye shall have them.

—Mark 11:23-24

Overcoming Temptation—

She looketh well to the ways of her household, and eateth not the bread of idleness.

—Proverbs 31:27

There hath no temptation taken you but such as is common to man; but God is faithful, who will not suffer you to be tempted above that ye are able; but will with the temptation also make a way to escape, that ye may be able to bear it.

—I Corinthians 10:13

For in that he himself hath suffered being tempted, he is able to succour them that are tempted.

—Hebrews 2:18

Let no man say when he is tempted, I am tempted of God: for God cannot be tempted with evil, neither tempteth he any man: But every man is tempted, when he is drawn away of his own lust, and enticed.

—James 1:13-14

Disciplining Yourself—

And every man that striveth for the mastery is temperate in all things. Now they do it to obtain a corruptible crown; but we an incorruptible. I therefore so run, not as uncertainly; so fight I, not as one that beateth the air; But I keep under my body, and bring it into subjection: lest that by any means, when I have preached to others, I myself should be a castaway.

—I Corinthians 9:25-27

Finally, brethren, whatsoever things are true, whatsoever things are honest, whatsoever things are just, whatsoever things are pure, whatsoever things are lovely, whatsoever things are of good report; if there be any virtue, and if there be any praise, think on these things.

—Philippians 4:8

APPENDIX II
Weight Charts

DESIRABLE WEIGHTS in pounds for adult men and women, according to height and frame, in light (summer) indoor clothing with pockets empty and no shoes.

Men Aged Twenty-five and Over

Height	Small Frame	Medium Frame	Large Frame
5 1	112—120	118—129	126—141
5 2	115—123	121—133	129—144
5 3	118—126	124—136	132—148
5 4	121—129	127—139	135—152
5 5	123—133	130—143	138—156
5 6	128—137	134—147	142—161
5 7	132—141	138—152	147—166
5 8	136—145	142—156	151—170
5 9	140—150	146—160	155—174
5 10	144—154	150—165	159—179
5 11	148—158	154—170	164—184
6 0	152—162	158—175	168—189
6 1	156—167	162—180	173—194
6 2	160—171	167—185	178—199
6 3	164—175	172—190	182—204

Women Aged Twenty-five and Over

Height	Small Frame	Medium Frame	Large Frame
4 8	92— 98	96—107	104—119
4 9	94—101	98—110	106—122
4 10	96—104	101—113	109—125
4 11	99—107	104—116	112—128
5 0	102—110	107—119	115—131
5 1	105—113	110—122	118—134
5 2	108—116	113—126	131—138
5 3	111—119	116—130	125—142
5 4	114—123	120—135	129—146
5 5	118—127	124—139	133—150
5 6	122—131	128—143	137—154
5 7	126—135	132—147	141—158
5 8	130—140	136—151	145—163
5 9	134—144	140—155	149—168
5 10	138—148	144—159	153—173

Young people between eighteen and twenty-five years, subtract one pound for each year under twenty-five. Consult pediatrician's charts for adolescents and children.

For nude weight, deduct three pounds for men and two pounds for women.

Weight charts used by courtesy of the Metropolitan Insurance Company.

APPENDIX III
Exercise Program For Men & Women

Judith A. Gray/Illustrator

WOMEN'S PROGRAM

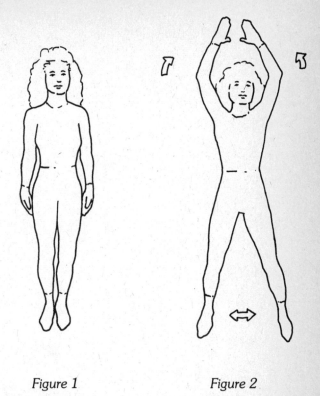

Figure 1   Figure 2

JUMPING JACKS— This exercise is for general toning up of the body. Begin standing straight with feet together, hands at sides *(Figure 1)*. Swing arms over head while spreading feet apart *(Figure 2)*. Return to starting position. Do set of twenty to begin exercise.

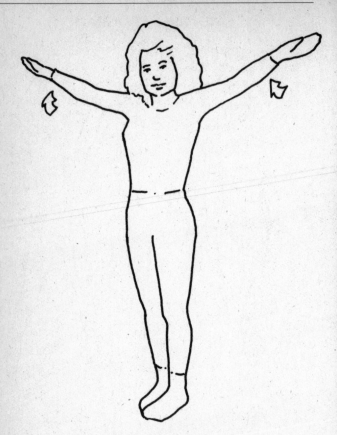

ARM CIRCLES— Stand with feet apart and arms straight out from shoulders. Begin by turning arms in small circles with palms down. Do set of ten and then reverse doing ten circles with palms up. Then repeat same procedure with medium circles and then big circles. Firms arms.

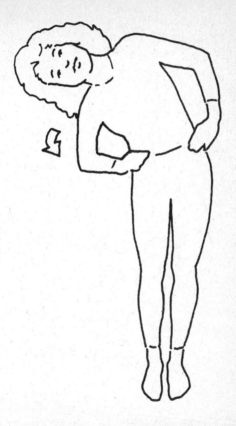

BODY ROTATION— Standing straight with hands on hips. Bend forward, then return to starting position. Then bend to the left, return, bend back, return, and bend to the right and return. Do sets of ten. Firms waist.

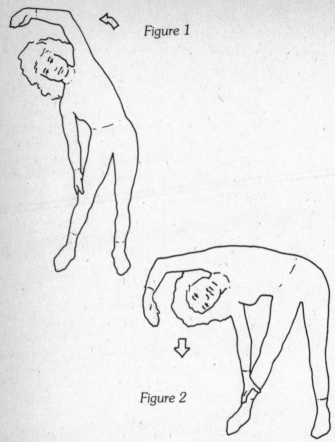

Figure 1

Figure 2

BODY STRETCH— Standing straight with feet apart and left arm above head and right arm at the side, stretch right arm (and body) to touch knee *(Figure 1)*. Do set of five on each side. Then repeat extending arm down to ankle *(Figure 2)*. Firms hips.

Figure 1

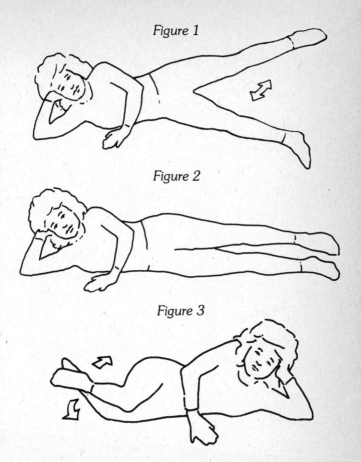

Figure 2

Figure 3

SCISSOR KICK— Lying on side in prone position, lift legs six inches off floor *(Figure 1)*. Scissor legs in set of fifty *(Figure 2)*. Repeat same with bicycle leg motion *(Figure 3)*. Firms legs and thighs.

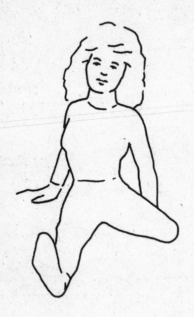

HIP & THIGH SLIMMER— Sit on floor with left foot extended and right leg curled back. Grasp right foot with right hand. Twist hips, hold ten seconds. Repeat on other side. Repeat ten times. Firms hips.

MEN'S PROGRAM
For Shoulder, Arm and Chest Strength

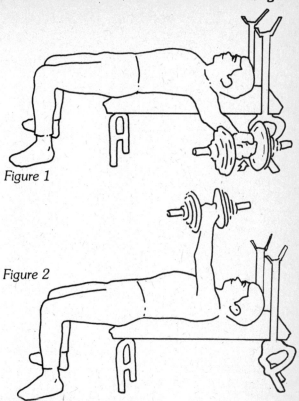

Figure 1

Figure 2

SIDE PRESS— Lie flat on back on floor or bench. Using 5 to 40 pound dumb-bell*, start exercise with arm extended straight out to side *(Figure 1)*. Lift dumb-bell, bringing arm to position directly above chest *(Figure 2)* and then slowly back to extended position. Do 3 sets of 8-10.

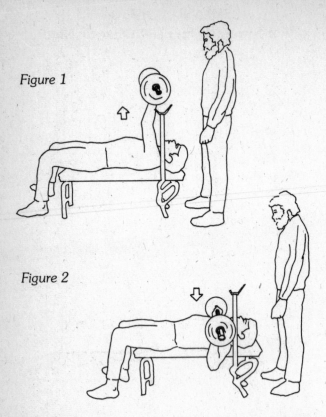

Figure 1

Figure 2

BENCH PRESS— Lying flat on back with bar-bell*
across chest, lift barbell straight up until arms are fully extended *(Figure 1)*. Bend elbows until barbell comes down
to within 3 inches of chest *(Figure 2)*. Lift to extended
position. Do 3 sets of 8-10. For safety precautions, a
standby person should always be present when bench
pressing weights.

Figure 1

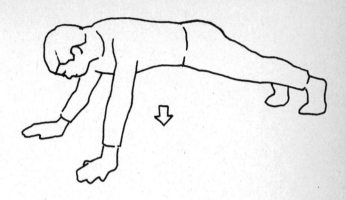

Figure 2

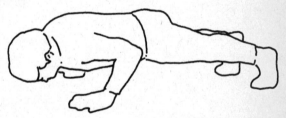

PUSH-UPS— Push-ups may be done in place of and/or in addition to the bench press. Begin in prone position, legs and arms straight *(Figure 1)*. Bend arms until nose touches floor *(Figure 2)* and push back up to starting position. Repeat as many times as possible, increasing by one every other workout until you can do 30 at once.

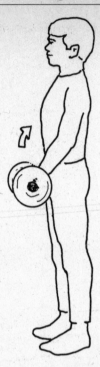

CURLS— Using either dumb-bells or bar-bell*, start with arms extended in front of hips. Curl arm up to chest then return to starting position. Do 3 sets of 8-10.

*The amout of weight used in these exercises depends on the person and the person's goal in the exercise. In order to build strength, use maximum weight which enables you to do only 8 to 10 repetitions without rest. To build endurance, use lighter weights but do more repetitions - 15 to 20.

Stomach Strength

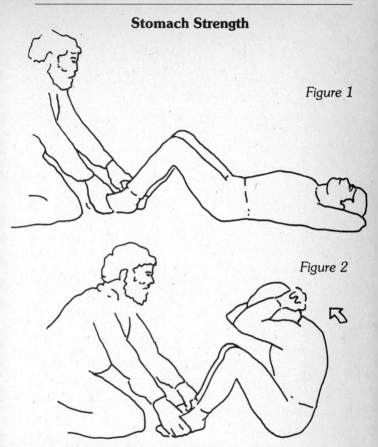

Figure 1

Figure 2

SIT-UPS— Lie on back with knees bent (legs fully extended can be harmful to the back); place hands behind head *(Figure 1)*. Sit up until chest touches knees *(Figure 2)*. Repeat as many times as possible, increasing by 2 sit-ups every third workout.

Figure 1

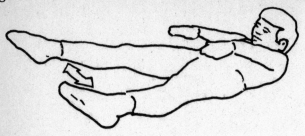

Figure 2

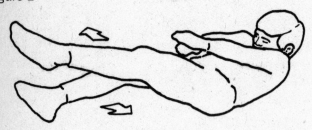

CROSS OVERS— Lie on back with arms and legs fully extended. Raise back until shoulders are six inches off floor with hands over legs. Lift feet six inches off floor *(Figure 1)*. Separate arms and legs, then bring them toward each other, crossing them as they come together *(Figure 2)*. Do two sets of twenty.

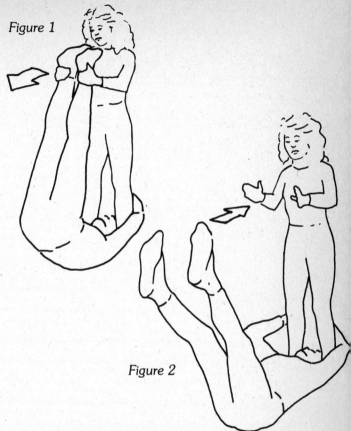

Figure 1

Figure 2

LEG THROW —Lie on back with legs straight. Lift legs to ninety degree angle. Partner throws legs back toward floor *(Figure 1)*. With stomach muscles, resist this push, not letting heels touch floor *(Figure 2)*. As legs return to starting position, partner throws them again. Repeat 15-20 times.

Legs and Calf Muscle Strength

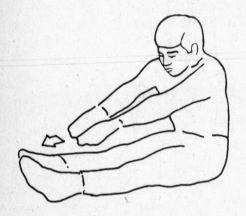

TOE TOUCHES— Begin in sitting position with legs extended. Extend arms forward individually to touch opposite toe. Do not bounce but extend slowly and steadily. Bouncing can cause strained or pulled muscles.

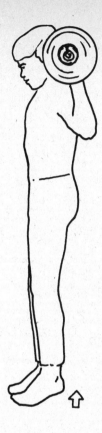

HEEL RAISES— Place bar-bell squarely on shoulders, balancing it with both hands. Begin with heels squarely on floor. Raise heels as high as possible and then back to floor. Repeat twenty times. Remember to have partner stand by on this exercise.

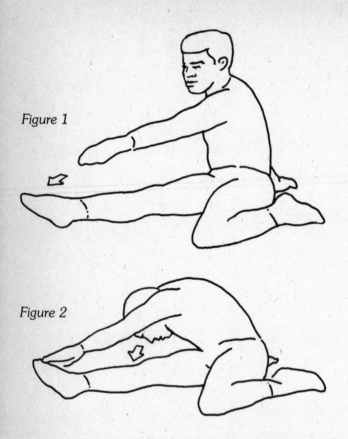

Figure 1

Figure 2

HURDLE STRETCH— Begin with one leg fully extended, other leg curled under body *(Figure 1)*. With opposite arm (from extended leg) touch extended toe bringing head down toward knee *(Figure 2)*. Repeat twenty times.

Figure 1   *Figure 2*

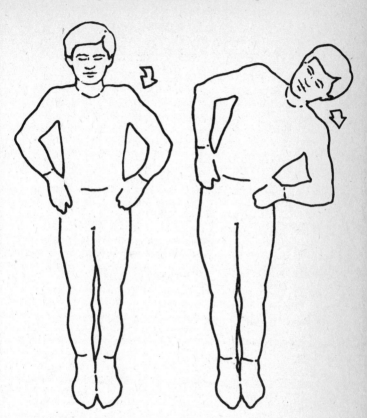

BODY ROTATION— In standing position with legs slightly apart, rotate body trunk *(Figure 1)*. First lean forward, then to the left side *(Figure 2)*, then backwards, then to the right side, then return to the starting position. Repeat twenty times.

APPENDIX IV
Aerobics Exercise Plan

Below is an exercise program designed to maintain a proper physical fitness level for anyone as suggested by the Aerobics plan. Points/week refer to the value of exercise to the body — 30 point minimum/week is suggested. Notice fitness level can be maintained by exercising only 15-60 minutes, 3 to 6 times a week.

Exercise Programs — Aerobics Plan

Fitness level is satisfactory—only requirement is to maintain fitness using one of the following programs:

	Distance (miles)	Time Goal (minutes)	Freq/wk	Points/wk
Running	1.0	under 8:00	6	30
	or 1.0	under 6:30	5	30
	or 1.5	under 12:00	4	30
	or 2.0	under 16:00	3	30
Swimming	(yards) 500	8:20-12:29	8	32
	or 600	10:00-14:59	6	30
	or 800	13:20-19:59	5	32
	or 1000	16:40-24:59	4	34
Cycling	(miles) 5.0	15:00-19:59	6	30
	or 6.0	18:00-23:59	5	30
	or 8.0	24:00-31:59	4	32
	or 10.0	30:00-39:59	3	30
Walking	(miles) 2.0	24:00-29:00	8	32
	or 3.0	36:00-43:30	5	30
	or 4.0	48:00-58:00	4	32
	or 5.0	60:00-72:30	3	30

	Duration (min.)	Freq (steps/min.)		
Stationary Running	10:00 in a.m & 10:00 in p.m.	70−80 70−80	5	30
	or 15:00	70−80	7	30
	or 15:00	80−90	5	30
	or 20:00	80−90	4	32

	Time (min.)*	Freq/wk	Points/wk
Handball Squash Basketball	40	5	30
	or 50	4	30
	or 70	3	30

*Continuous exercise. Do not count breaks, etc.

APPENDIX V
Diet Food Recipes

Granola

6	Cups	Rolled Oats
1	Cup	Wheat Germ
½	Cup	Chopped Walnuts
½	Cup	Sliced Almonds
½	Cup	Coconut
½	Cup	Sunflower Seeds (or more)
¾	Cup	Honey
½	Cup	Vegetable Oil

Heat oats and wheat germ on a pan at 350° for 10 minutes. Combine honey and oil, set aside. Combine all other ingredients and add oats and wheat germ. Pour honey and oil mixture over it and mix thoroughly. Spread evenly in pan and bake at 350° for 20-25 minutes stirring often (especially toward the end or it will burn.) Cool and stir. Add raisins and/or dates.

Honey Wheat Bread

1½	Cups	Water
1	Cup	Cottage Cheese
½	Cup	Honey
¼	Cup	Margarine
4½-5	Cups	All Purpose Flour
2	Cups	Wheat Flour
2	Tblsp.	Sugar
3	Tsp.	Salt
2	Pkg.	Dry Yeast
1		Egg

Heat first four ingredients until very warm. Combine this warm liquid with 2 Cups Flour and remaining ingredients. Beat 2 minutes. Stir in remaining flour to make stiff dough. Knead until smooth and elastic. Put in greased bowl and let rise until double. Punch down and divide into two loaves or 24 rolls. Let rise again till double. Bake at 350° till golden brown and sounds hollow to tap. Brush the warm loaves with honey and butter mix.

APPENDIX VI
Jim Bakker's Diet Plan

MENU

BREAKFAST—

One (1) Large Serving of Whole Grain Cereal — Use recipe in Appendix V or purchase at a Health Food Store. Make sure there are no sugar additives.

A Variety of Fresh Fruit — Apples, pears, oranges, bananas — If canned goods are used, make sure the food is not canned in heavy syrup. Use food that is canned in its natural juices. You may have to get it in the dietetic section of your grocery store.

A Variety of Vegetables — Always undercook rather than overcook vegetables to retain the natural vitamins and minerals. All vegetables should be prepared by steaming.

A Variety of Fruit Juices — Orange, grapefruit, prune — Be sure there are no sugar additives.

NOTE: Use one percent (1%) fat in milk on cereal, or skimmed milk if you prefer.

I recommend doing exercises before breakfast. I feel, this way, you burn up fat that has been stored in the body.

LUNCH —

One (1) Small Piece of Meat — Lean Beef (Because of animal fat content, try not to eat more than three times a week.), baked poultry, lamb, or broiled seafood. Stay away from pork and forbidden foods in the Old Testament for health's sake.

A Variety of Vegetables — Vegetables should always be steamed.

A Variety of Fruit —

Salad — No dressing — You may use plain vinegar or lemon juice.

DINNER —

One (1) Small Piece of Meat — Same as for lunch.

A Variety of Vegetables — Same as for lunch.

A Variety of Fruit — Same as for lunch.

NOTE: To satisfy that hunger craving, I would suggest Chinese food. However, stay away from all fried foods and order the dishes that are prepared with sprouts and vegetables, for instance, Chicken Chow mein.

Stay away from fast-food chains.

"No-No's" for the first two months: soft drinks unless artificially sweetened; breads unless specifically recommended health breads; desserts of all kinds.

APPENDIX VII
Test for Hypoglycemia

Self-Check Questions for Hypoglycemia

This questionaire lists every possible hypoglycemia symptom, and ask patients to mark any and all symptoms they've experienced. To use it yourself, mark the number "1" next to the symptoms or characteristics you experience mildly, "2" for somewhat strongly, and "3" for severely. When you've finished, add up the figures. Any total above 20 reveals the need of a glucose test by a qualified physician.

1. _____ Craving for sweets
2. _____ Craving for candy or coffee in afternoons
3. _____ Craving for alcohol
4. _____ Great consumption of coffee as a pick-me-up
5. _____ Eat often, otherwise get hunger pains or faintness
6. _____ Eat when nervous
7. _____ Hunger between meals
8. _____ "Shaky" when hungry
9. _____ Faintness when meals delayed
10. _____ Fatigue that is relieved by eating
11. _____ Heart palpitations when meals missed or delayed
12. _____ Irritability before meals
13. _____ Sleepy after meals
14. _____ Sleepy during day
15. _____ Feel better after breakfast than before
16. _____ Awaken after few hours sleep—hard to get back to sleep
17. _____ Anxious dreams
18. _____ Afternoon headaches
19. _____ "Butterfly" stomach, cramps

20. _____ Inability to get started in morning before coffee
21. _____ Allergies—tendency to asthma, hay fever, skin rash, etc.
22. _____ Heavy breathing
23. _____ Bleeding gums
24. _____ Spotting or bronzing of skin
25. _____ Blurred vision
26. _____ Inability to make decisions
27. _____ Inability to work under pressure
28. _____ Chronic fatigue
29. _____ Chronic nervous exhaustion
30. _____ Lack of energy
31. _____ Lack of initiative
32. _____ Cry easily for no reason
33. _____ Weakness, dizziness
34. _____ Convulsions
35. _____ Nervous trembling
36. _____ Hand tremors
37. _____ Highly emotional
38. _____ Fearful
39. _____ Hallucinations
40. _____ Dizziness
41. _____ Depression
42. _____ Insomnia
43. _____ Magnify insignificant events
44. _____ Poor memory
45. _____ Worry, feel insecure
46. _____ Moody or melancholy

I will not hesitate to emphasize the flaws in this type of diagnostic method, but it is valuable as a means for patients to recall and focus on any manifestations of their possible metabolic imbalances.

From *Nutrigenetics* by Dr. R. O. Brennan with William C. Mulligan. Copyright © 1975 by Richard O. Brennan. Reprinted by permission of the publisher M. Evans and Company, Inc., NY, NY 10017.

Medical Test for Hypoglycemia

The normal blood-sugar level is usually maintained between 80 and 120 mgs per 100 cc in people. In a healthy person this level neither rises much higher after a high-carbohydrate meal nor falls much lower after the usual twelve-hour fast from 7:00 pm to 7:00 am. Controlled quantities of insulin, released by the pancreas after a meal, cause any excess glucose to be stored in the liver and muscles, in the form of glycogen. This, in turn, is broken down again to glucose, during the night hours, to prevent the level from falling too low.

In the glucose-tolerance test, a drink containing 100 grams of glucose is given after a fast of several hours, and blood samples are taken from a vein at hourly intervals. The expected initial rise in blood glucose level during the first hour or two should soon start coming down to below 120 mgs. (If it does not, the patient probably has diabetes.)

With hypoglycemia or low blood sugar, the most typical curve is a drop to below 80 mgm usually at the 5th and 6th hour. Probably the more significant measurement is a drop of 20 points below the fasting level. This drop of 20 mgm below the fasting level may occur at any point during the six hour test. Another abnormal type of response with hypoglycemia is a totally flat curve in which the sugar neither rises nor falls from the fasting level. This is often associated with severe symptoms.